MW01623038

Let's Stay Connected.

Follow me on Social Media:

@jodigc

jodi.gc

Get Free Stuff:

Sign up at JodiCameron.com
to get your free gift.

Other books by Jodi Cameron:

Mind Monsters for Kids

FIGHT OF YOUR LIFE
by Jodi Cameron

Published by Spry Publishing
Issaquah, WA

Library of Congress Control Number: 2019907370

ISBN: 978-0-578-51278-5

Printed in USA

FAITH FOR YOUR FUTURE ***TODAY***

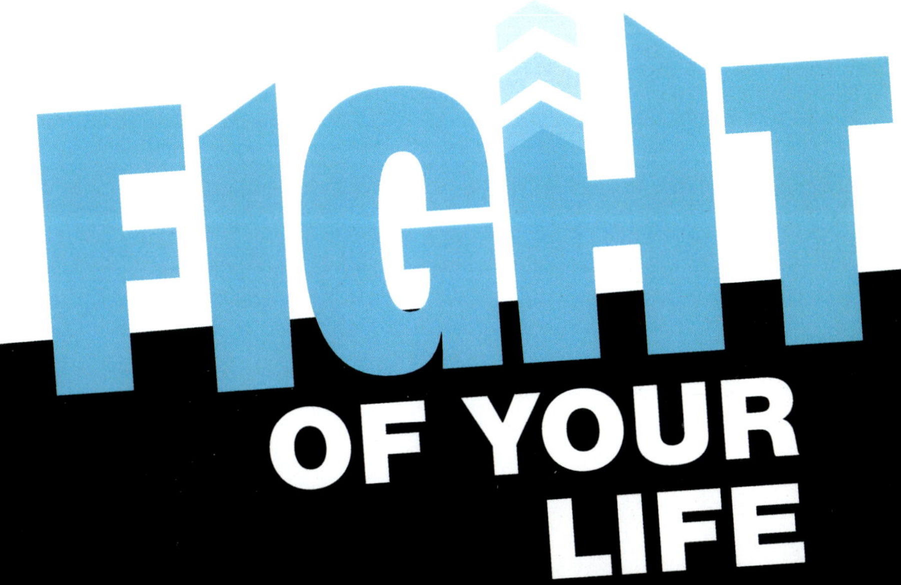

Dedicated to my parents, (Kevin & Sheila), for showing me what it is to fight the Good Fight.

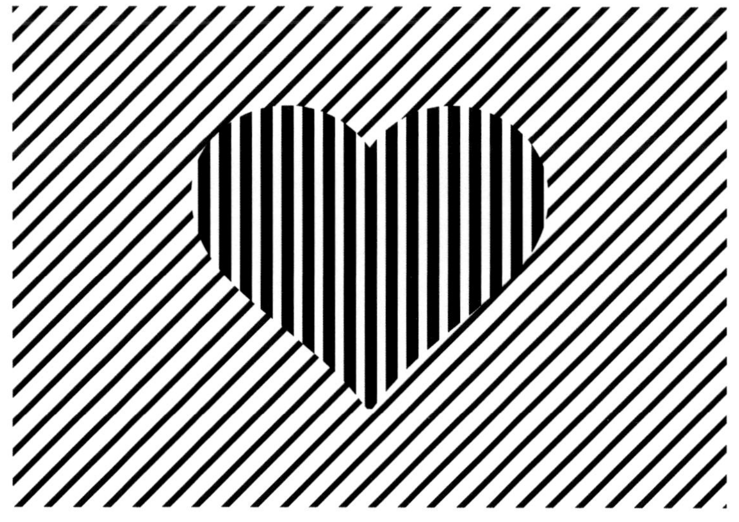

Thanks for fighting for good when everyone was watching, when only I was watching, and when only God was watching. I love you.

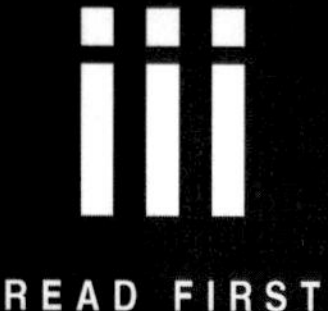

HEY FIGHT-ER!

THIS IS A
MINI BOOK
WITH A
MESSAGE.

YOU ARE A FIGHTER.

Yes, really, you are. And, I am. We were created to FIGHT. (That's why it comes so easily for most of us.) But, what if we learned how to FIGHT FOR our lives? What if we learned how to fight for what God wants in us? ... what He wants to do through us in our family... in our community... in our workplace... in our church? What if we changed how we fight?

What if we focused on what we are fighting for? (Instead of who we are fighting with...)

What if instead of fighting to be right, we chose to FIGHT FOR the absolute best in our life and relationships?

We can spend our energy on fighting to become the best version of ourselves, instead of using our energy to tear others down or taking control of every situation.

In the fight for your life, FIGHT FOR passion and purpose and God's best.

-Jodi

WE ARE

We all have a
fighter in us!

Are you **facing...**

A battle that looks impossible?

A battle that nobody believes you can win?

A battle that tests every ounce of faith you have?

NO MATTER WHAT BATTLE YOU ARE FACING OR WHAT FIGHT YOU ARE IN – **YOU** ARE NOT ALONE.

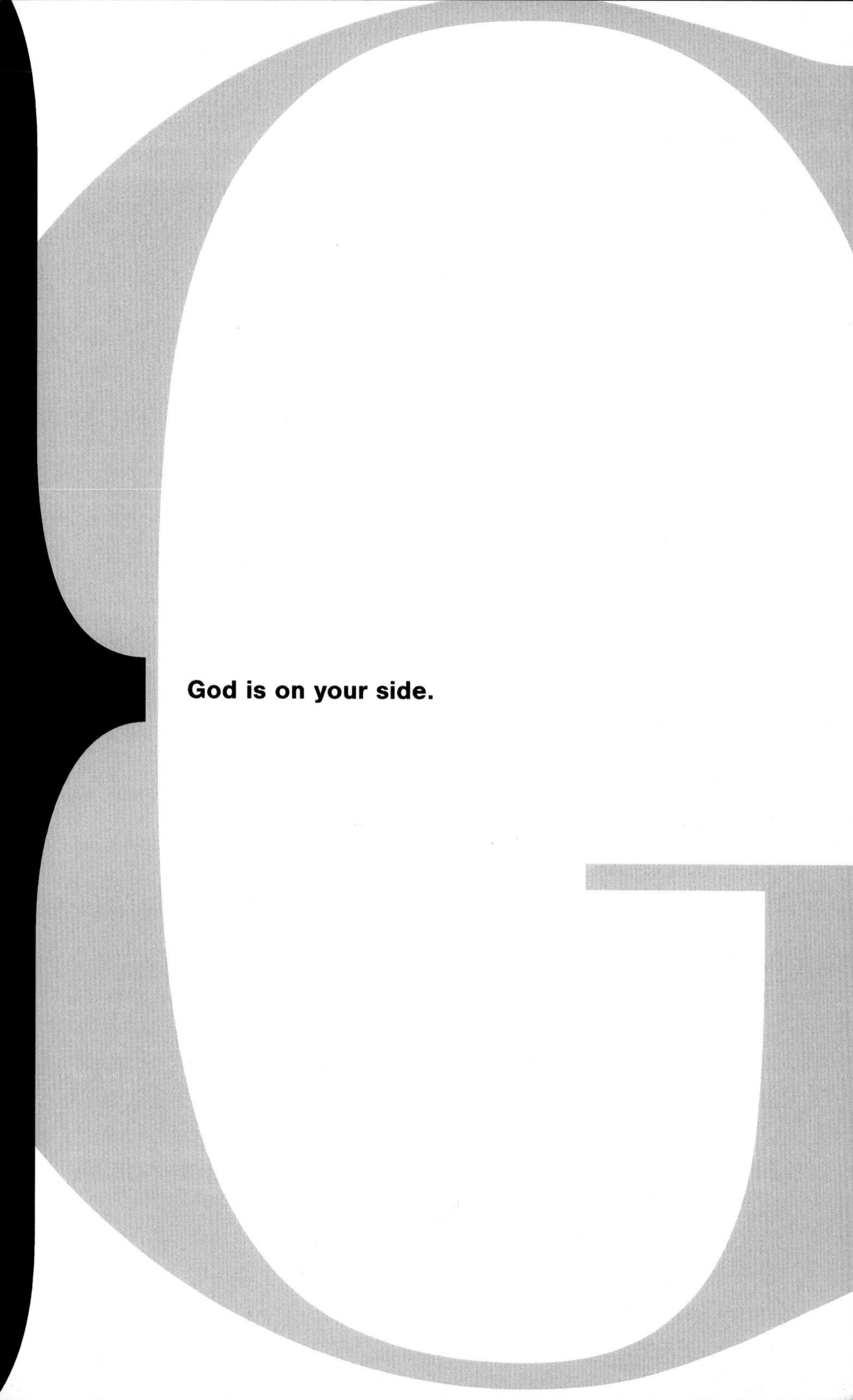

God is on your side.

YOU CAN WIN IF YOU DON'T QUIT

A WISE MENTOR ONCE TOLD A PROTÉGÉ TO

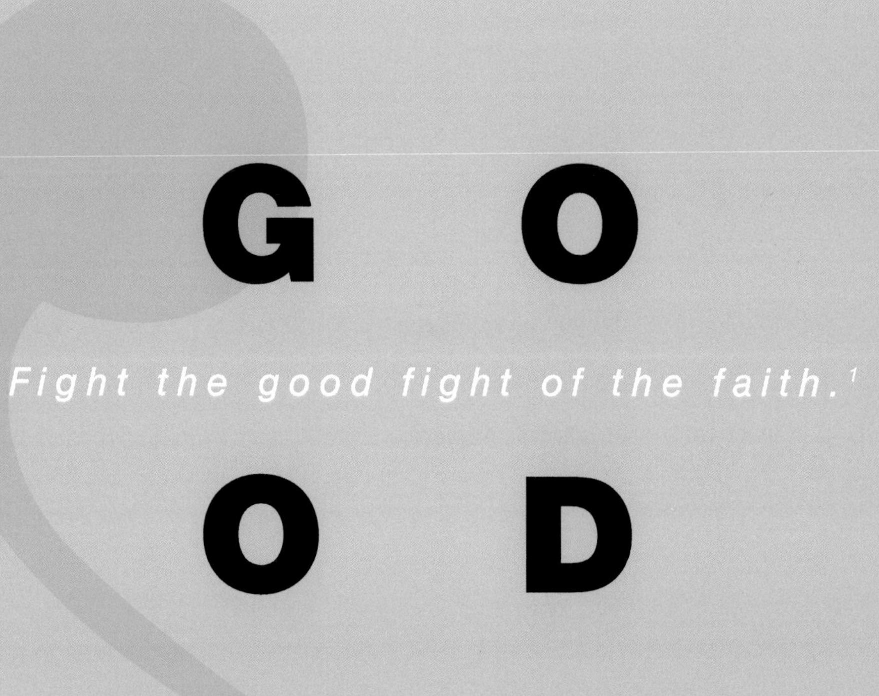

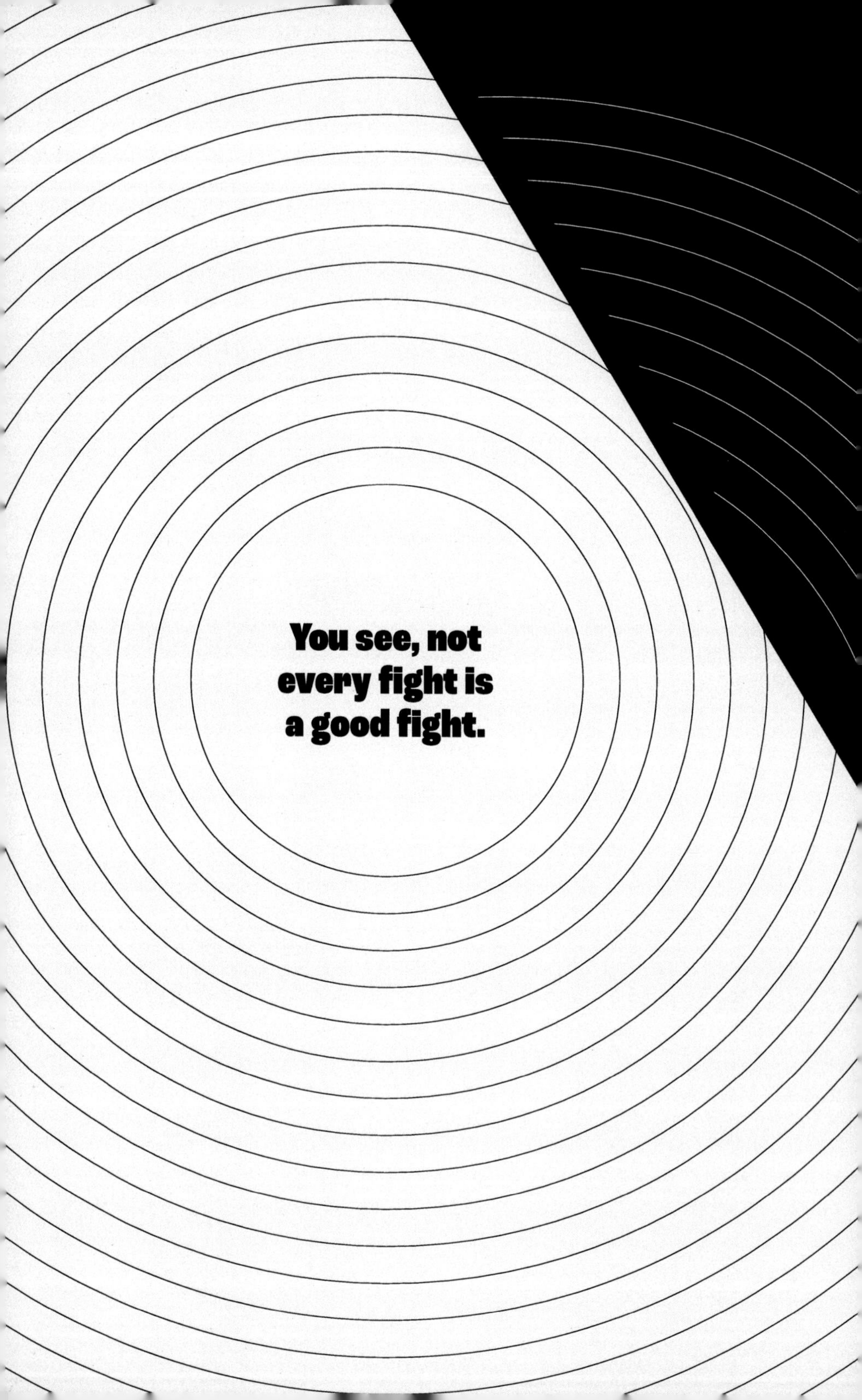
You see, not
every fight is
a good fight.

Sometimes,

we are fighting feelings, or perceptions, or assumptions. Some people just LOVE THE **FIGHT to be RIGHT.**

Not every fight is a good fight.

ok

Some fights aren't ours to fight.

And, that's ok.

Fighting the Good Fight

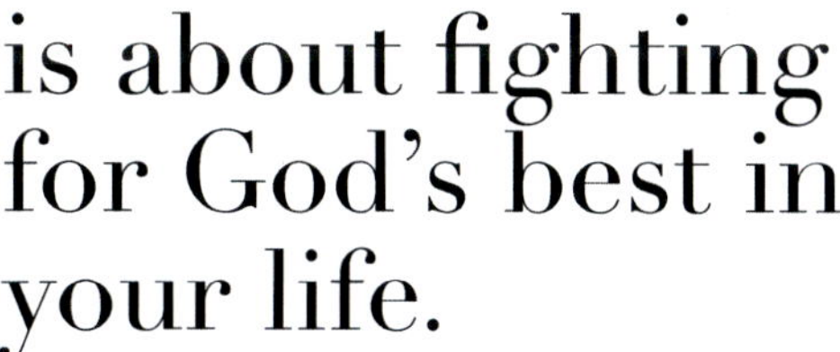

is about fighting for God's best in your life.

Imagine

what kind of future you want, the "God's best" version of your potential:

What does it ***look*** like?

What does it ***feel*** like?

Who does it ***include?***

Where is it ***happening?***

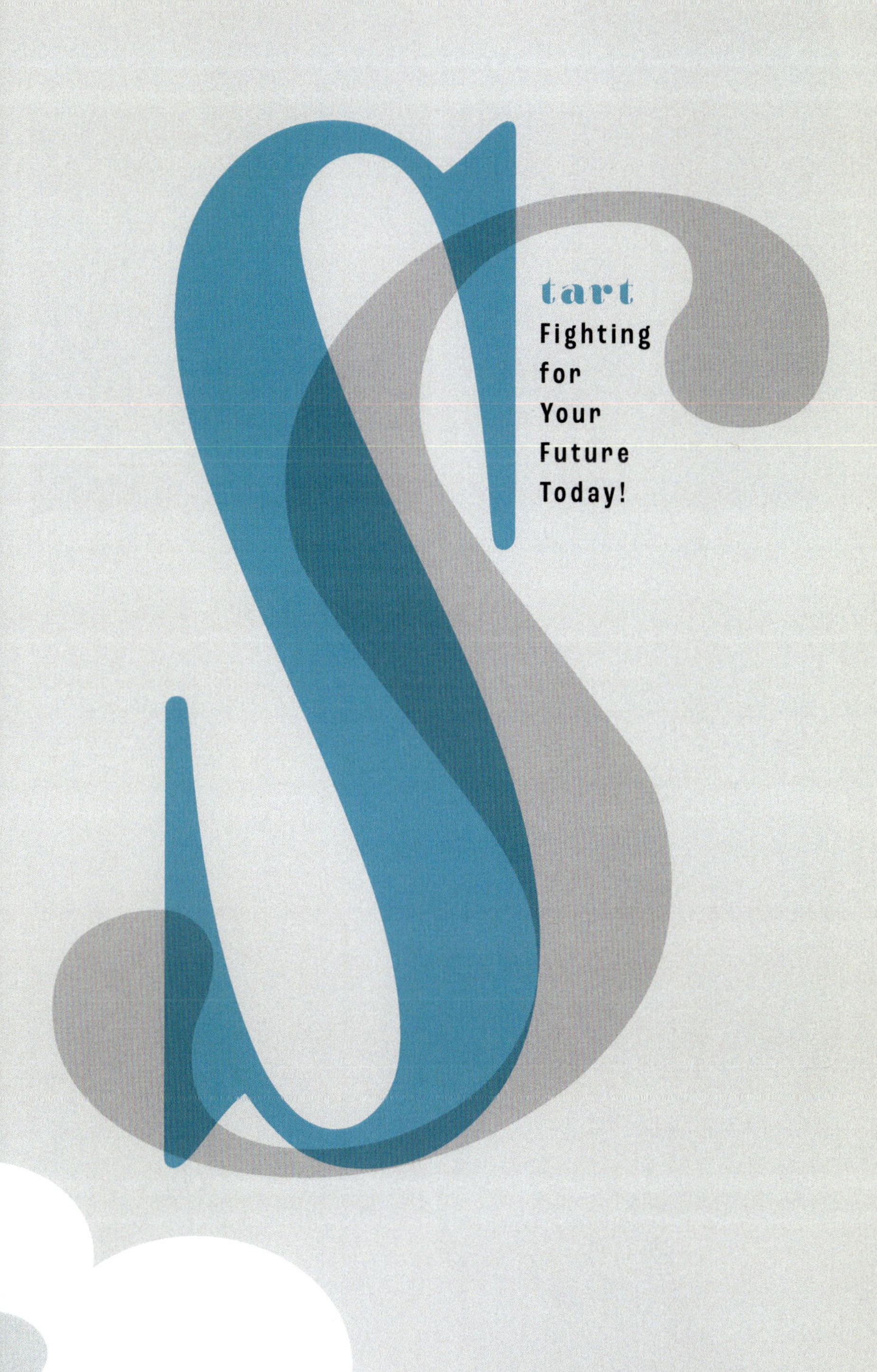
S
tart
Fighting
for
Your
Future
Today!

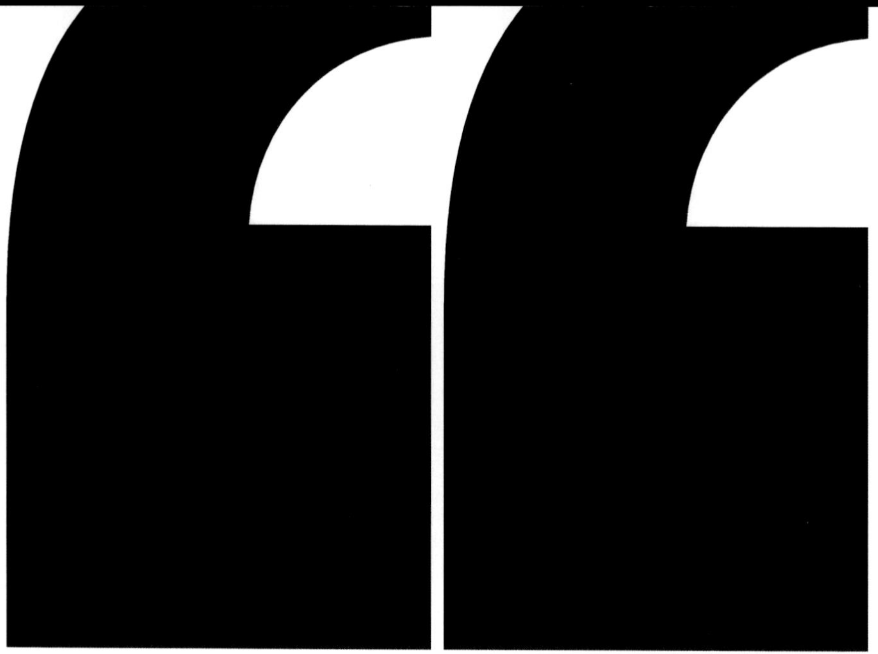

The decisions we make today will
impact our outcomes of tomorrow.[2]

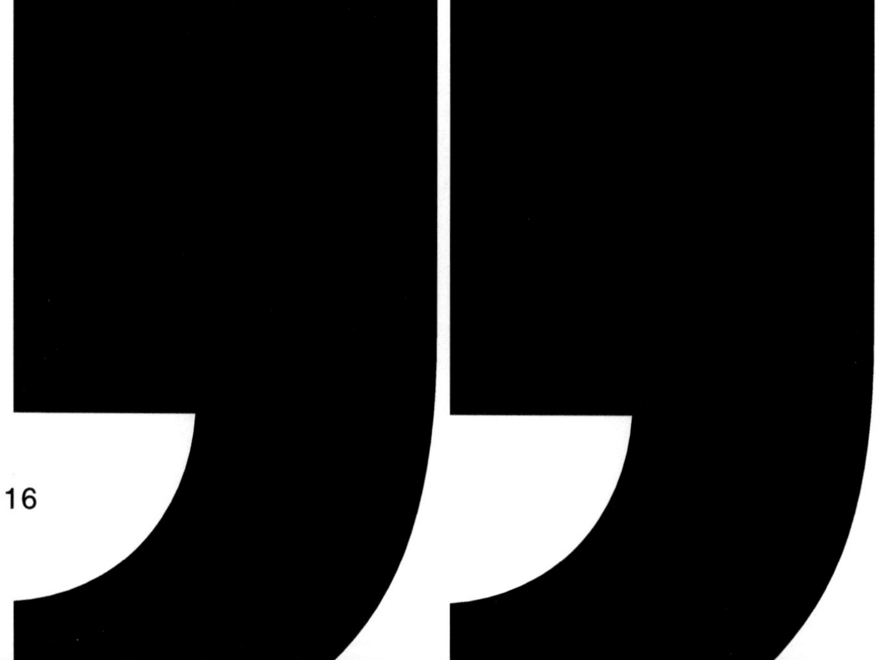

In fact, winning the battle of good decision making ***in the present*** *will only increase our ability for success in the future.*

YOU MAY BE IN THE FIGHT OF YOUR LIFE RIGHT NOW . . .

Fighting FOR joy,

Fighting FOR purity,

Fighting FOR health,

Fighting FOR love,

Fighting FOR purpose,

Fighting FOR family.

WHAT ARE YOU FIGHTING FOR?

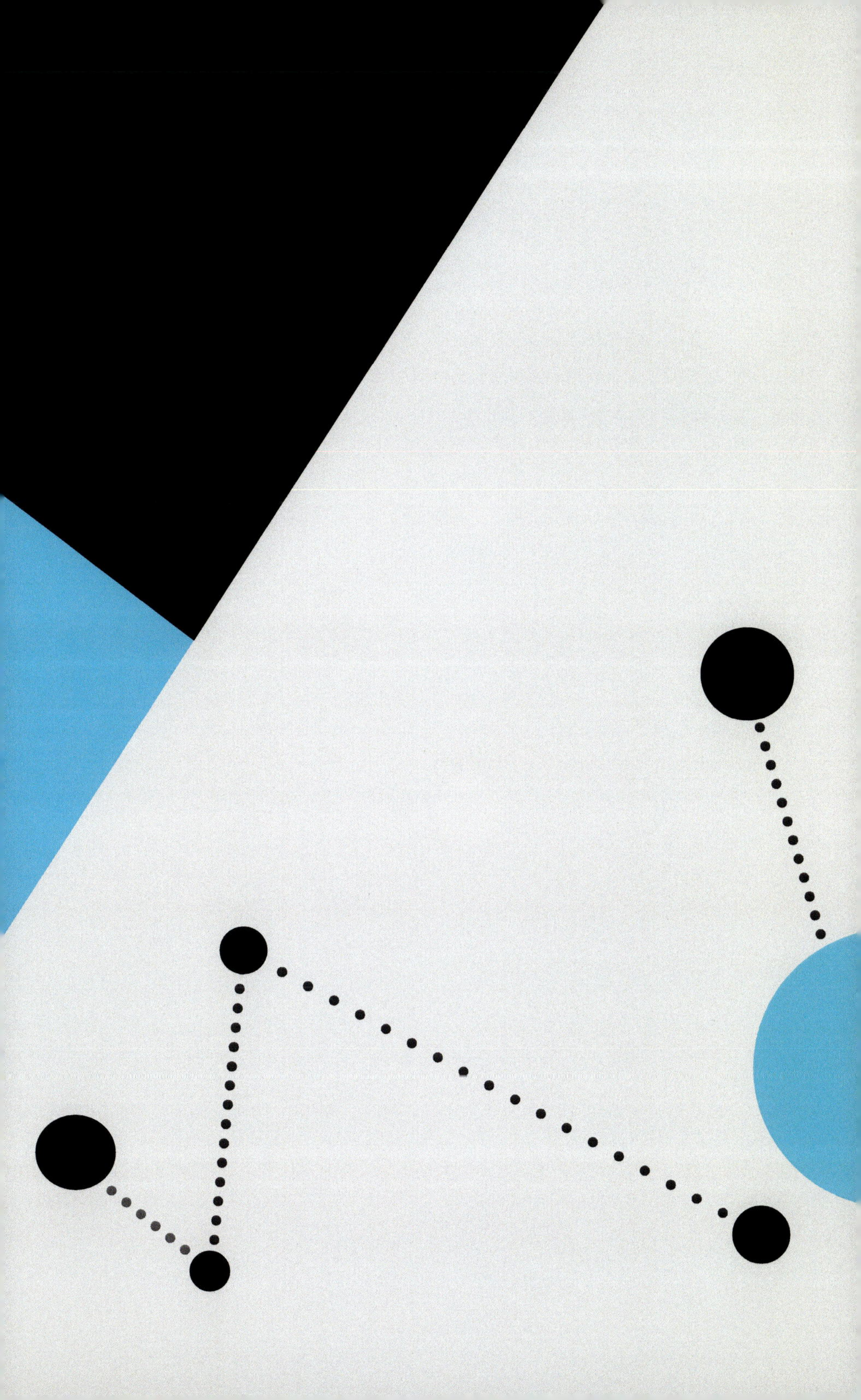

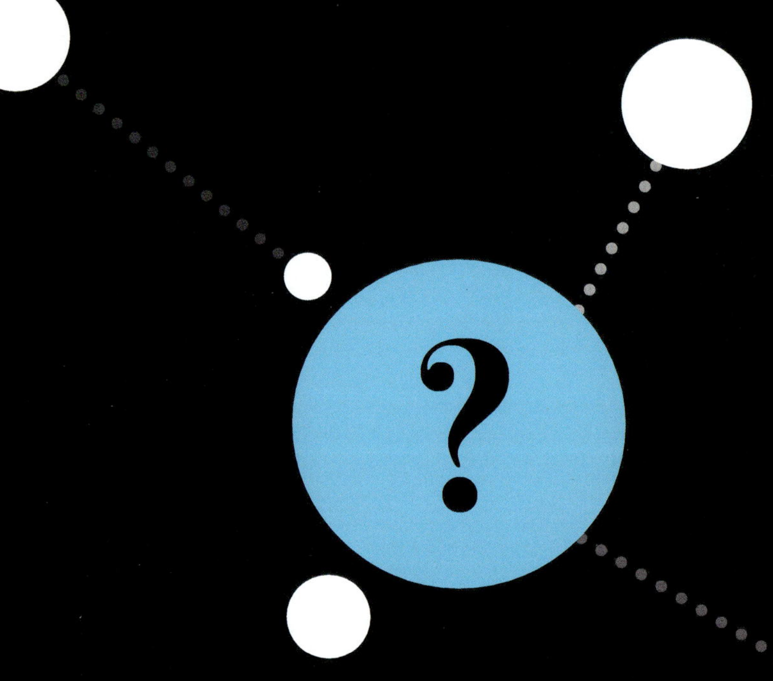

Ask Yourself:

Is this fight worth your energy?

Is it worth the investment needed?

Is this your fight to fight?

Does the price of the fight outweigh the prize of the fight?

If the price is

greater than

the prize, then it's time to

find a new fight.

LET'S BE THE KIND OF PEOPLE WHO FIGHT THE GOOD FIGHT.

We can fight for
God's best in
our lives!

HOW DO WE FIGHT THE GOOD FIGHT?

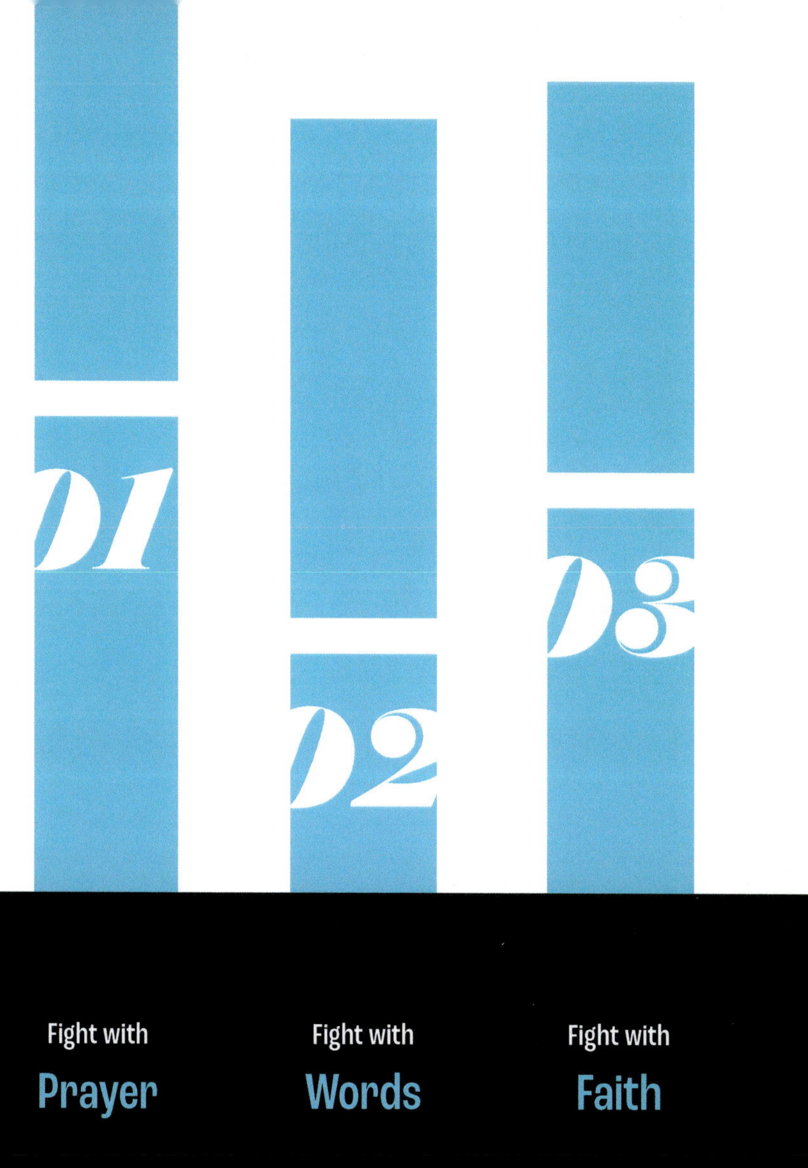

Fight with
Prayer

Fight with
Words

Fight with
Faith

FIGHT WITH PRAYER

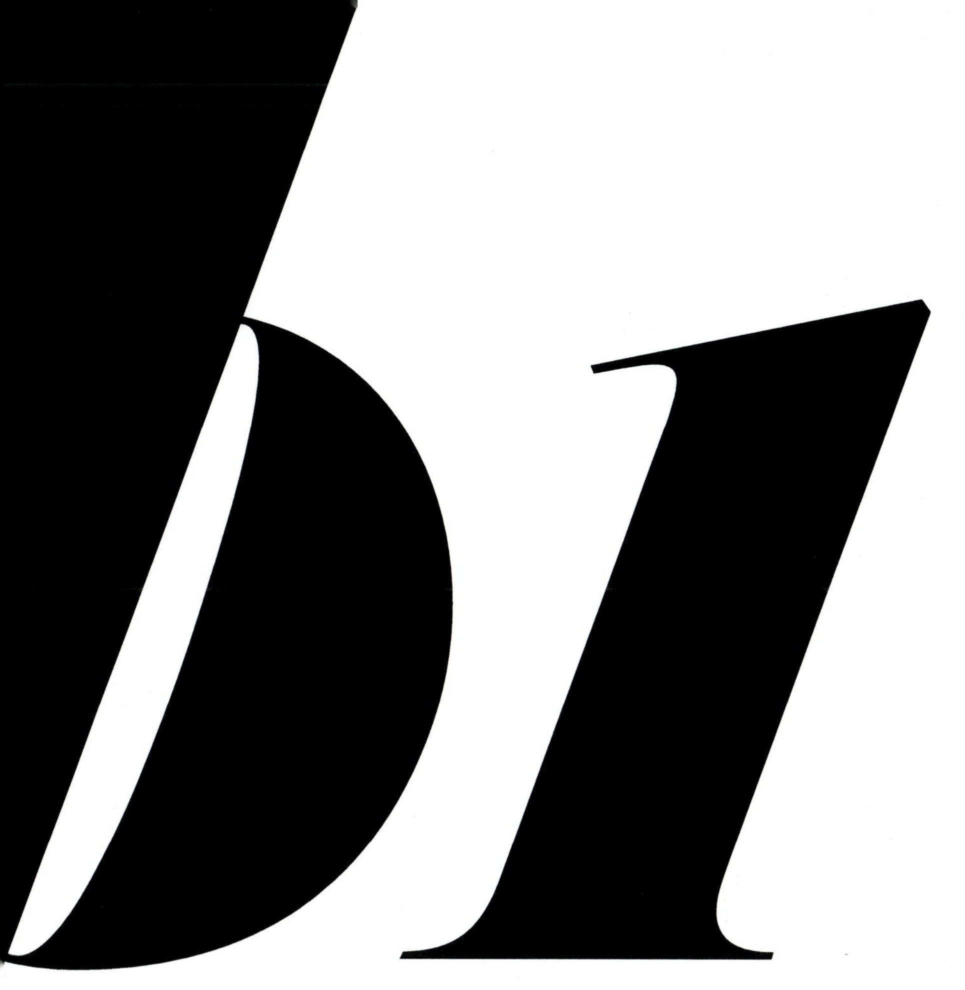

Prayer is important
in our everyday lives.
It doesn't have to be
complicated or flashy
or even eloquent.

prayer is simply

TALK ING

TO GOD

Just start talking to God throughout your day. Don't wait until you carve an hour of prayer into your day or until you have all the words right.

have an **ONGOING** *conversation with God* [3]

We won't always hear the audible voice of God. Sometimes, we may feel like our conversation with Him is one-sided. But, if we keep our eyes and ears and hearts open, God will speak to us.

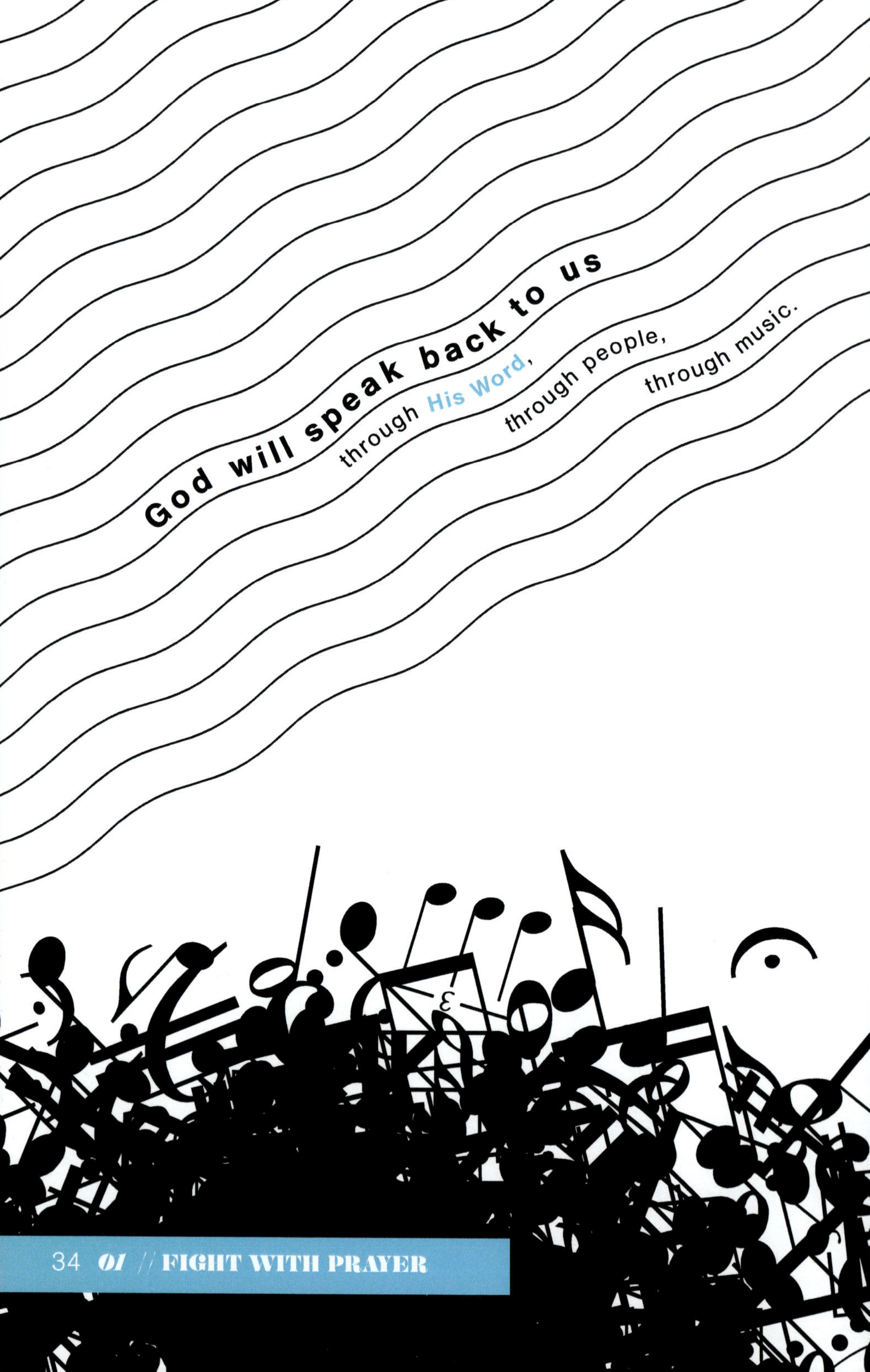
God will speak back to us
through His Word,
through people,
through music.

Assume God is listening when you pray and open up your heart to hear His response.

Prayer is
what changes
our circumstances.

And, if our circumstances are out of our control then prayer can still change **our perspective** about those circumstances.

FIGHT WITH WORDS

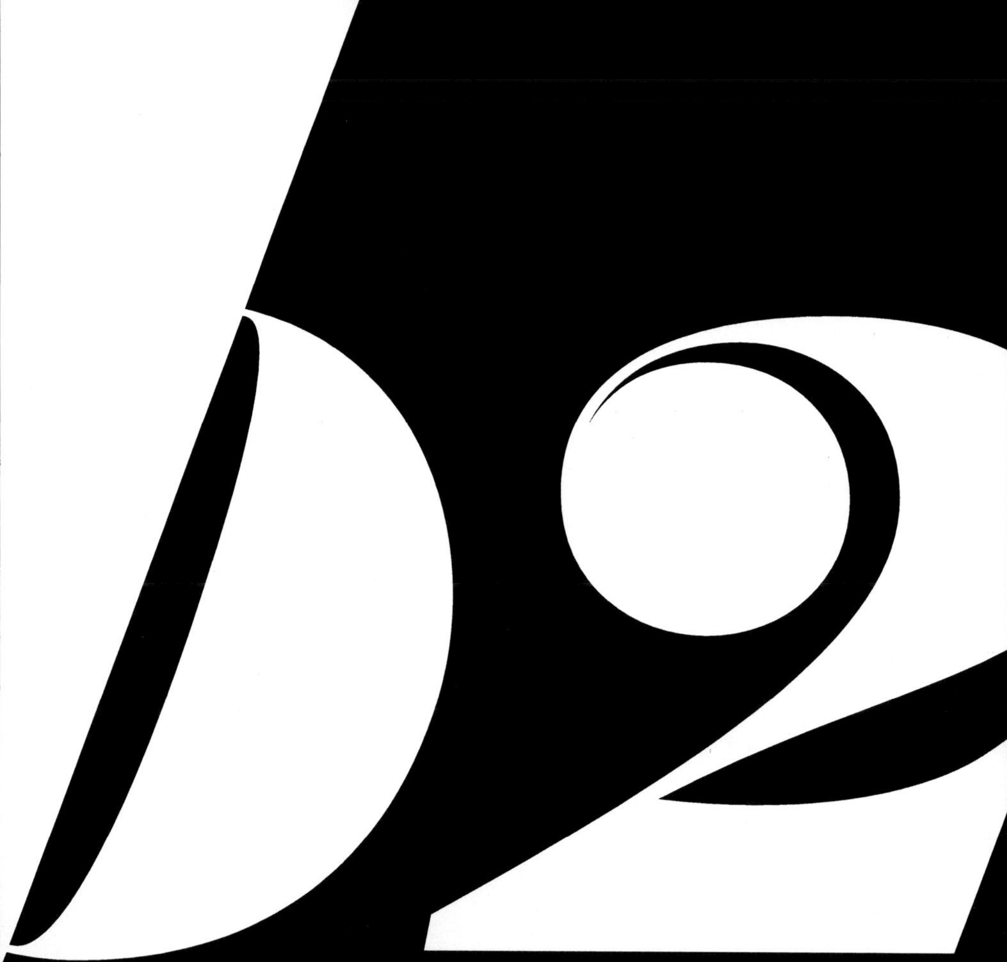

Words
can lift
you up

OR

words can
weigh you
down.

Words matter.

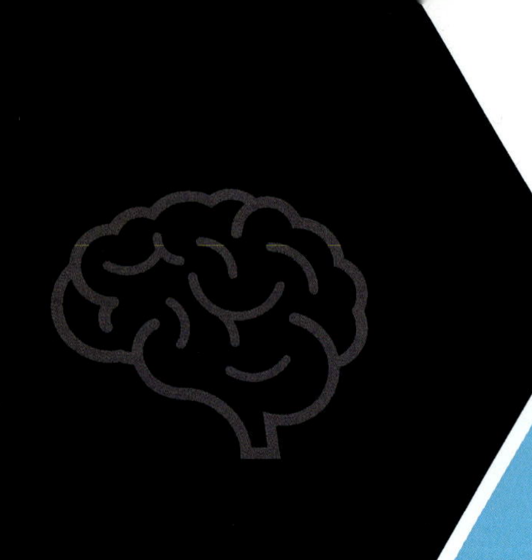

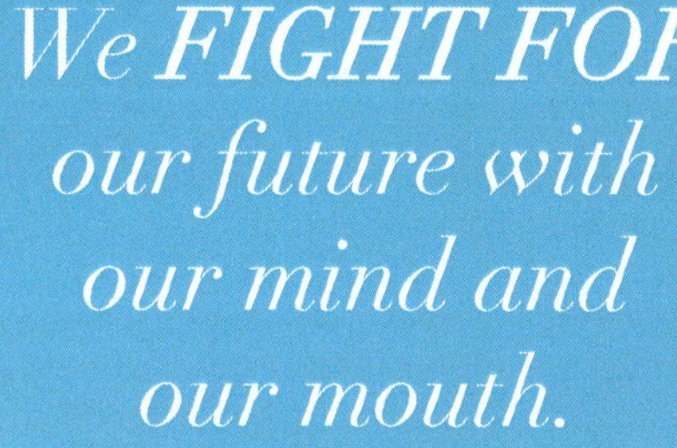

*We **FIGHT FOR** our future with our mind and our mouth.*

WHAT ARE YOU SAYING TO YOURSELF?

WHAT ARE YOU SAYING TO OTHERS?

WHAT WORDS DO YOU BELIEVE?

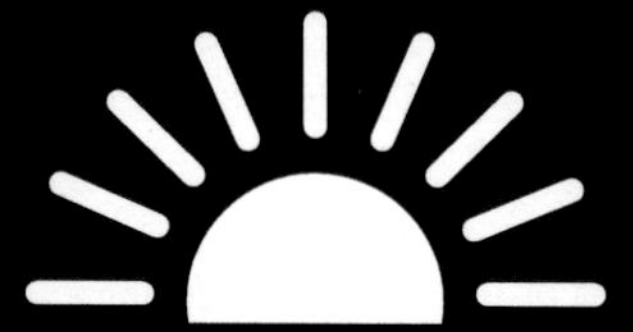

SPEAK TO BUILD YOURSELF UP.

■ ■ ■

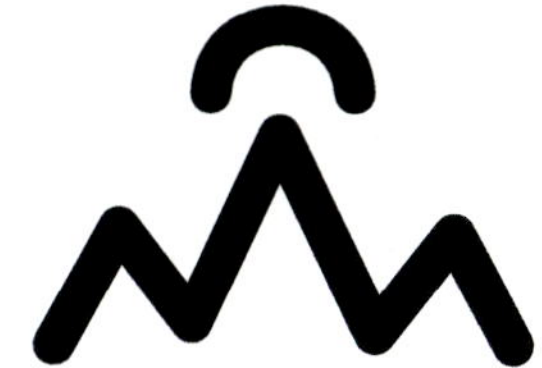

SPEAK TO YOUR FUTURE TODAY!

• • •

Harness the power of progress by creating a shift in your mindset: **speak positive** affirmations over your life.

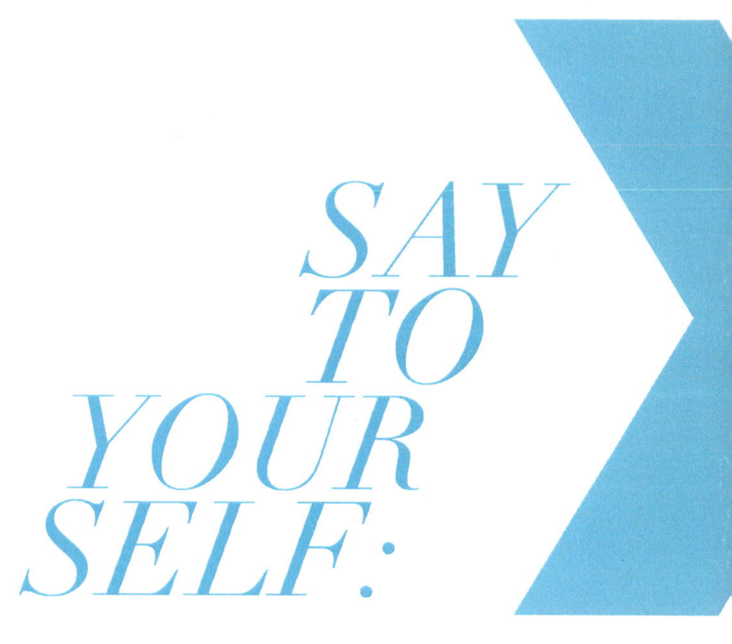
SAY
TO
YOUR
SELF:

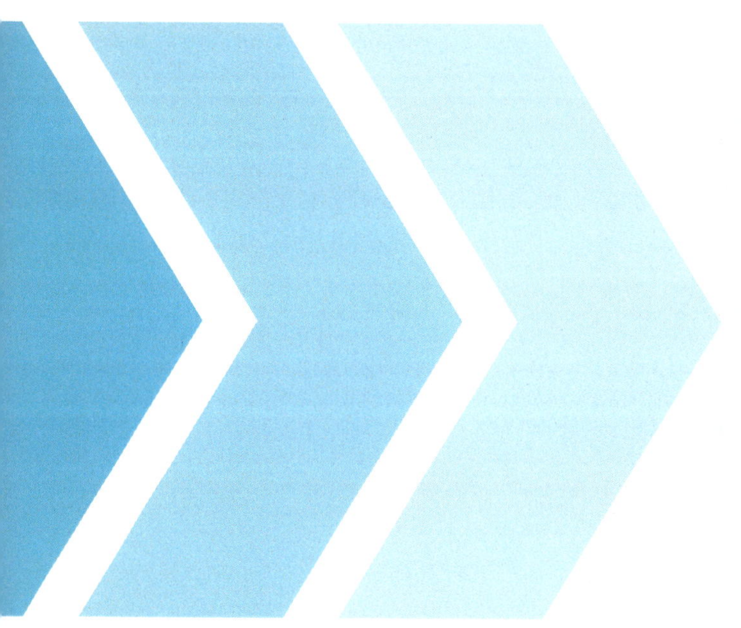

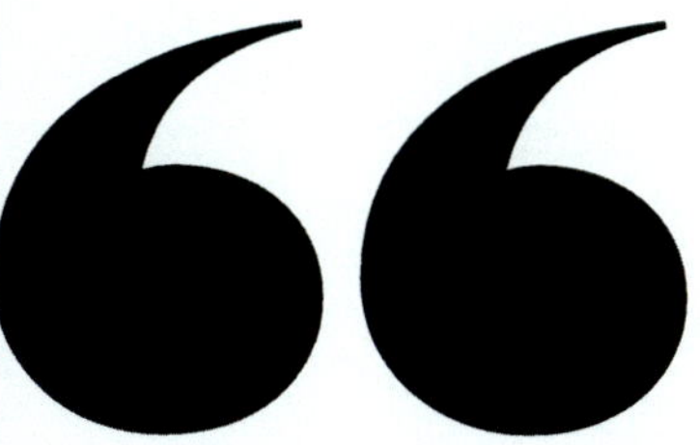

I am fantastic!

I am Godly.

I am flawed, yet God's grace is sufficient and thorough.

I am made whole and holy in God's love.

I have a purpose.

I walk with confidence everywhere I go.

I choose the ultimate over the immediate.

I am a child of The King.

I am surrounded by good things.

I choose attitudes today that will take me where I want to go tomorrow.

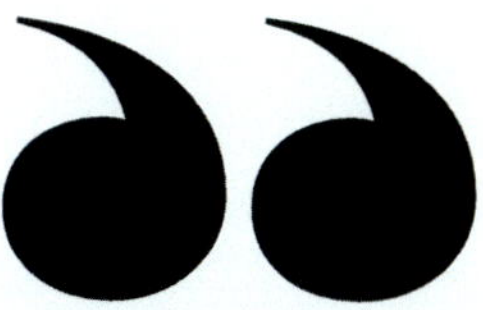

DON'T STOP WITH BUILDING YOURSELF UP, SPEAK TO BUILD OTHERS UP AS WELL!

And never let ugly or hateful words come from your mouth, but instead let your words become beautiful gifts that encourage others; do this by speaking words of grace to help them. [4]

FIGHT WITH FAITH

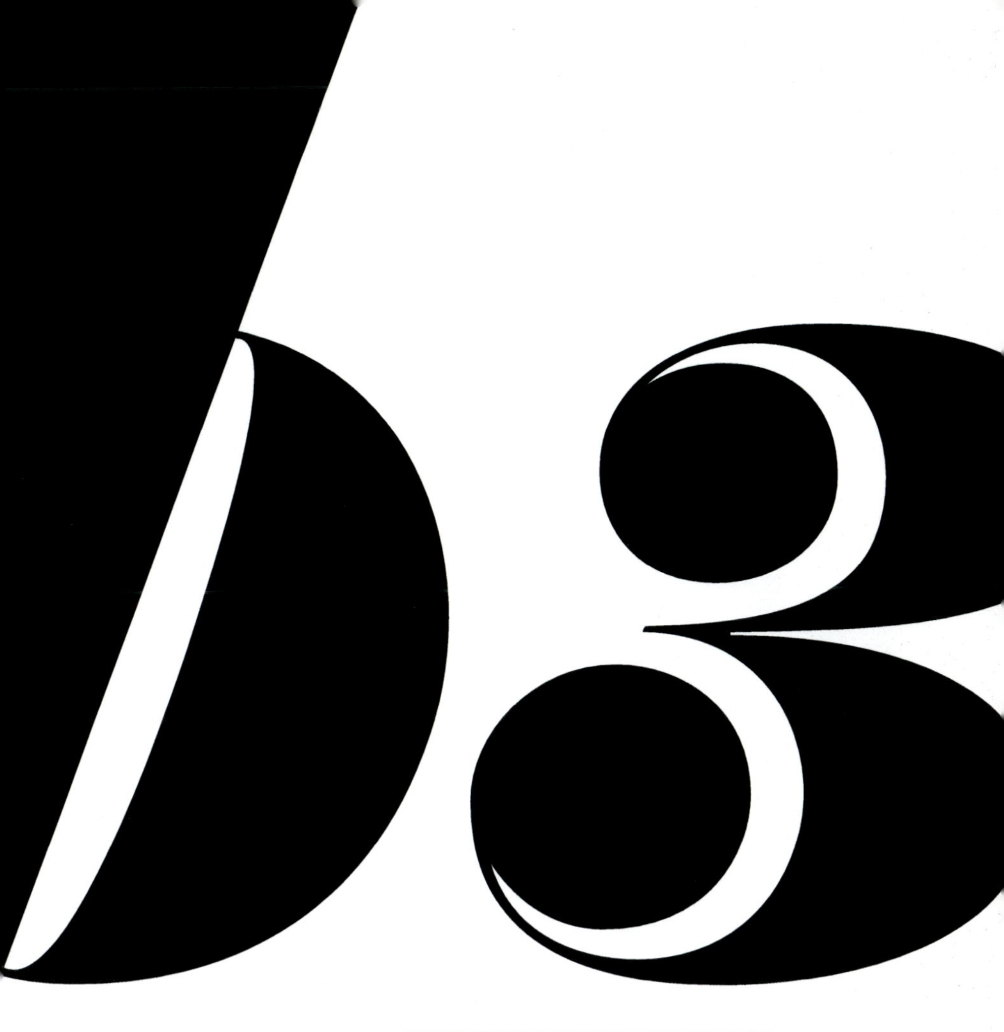

Fight for your future with FAITH and CONFIDENCE in the face of reality.

When we fight with faith, it means we put our trust in who God is and what He promises.

...It means

we take whatever the next step is to pursue God's best for our lives.

We do not have to know the end in order to begin.

We do not have to understand it all to move forward in FAITH.

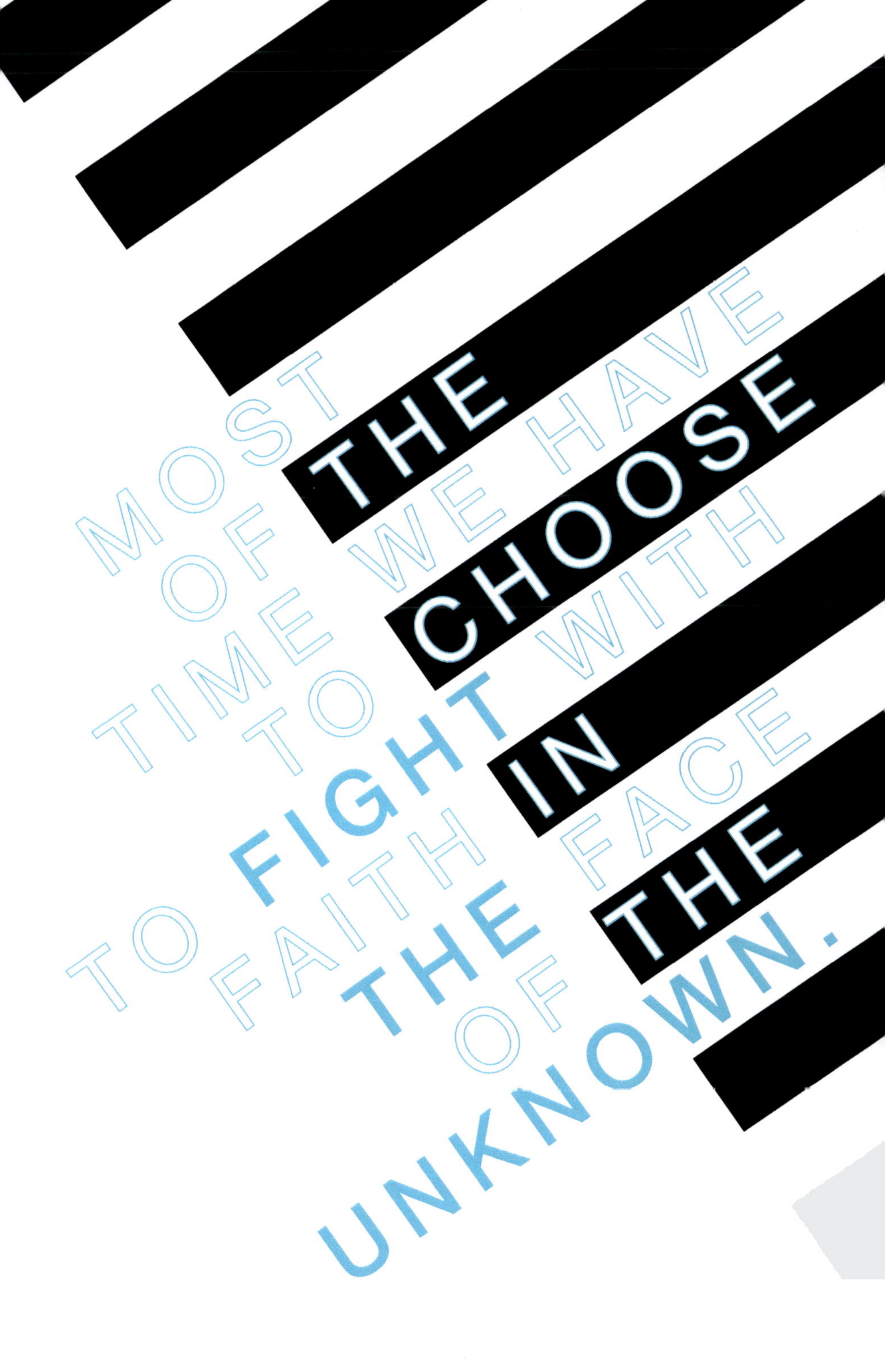
MOST OF THE TIME WE HAVE TO CHOOSE TO FIGHT WITH FAITH IN THE FACE OF THE UNKNOWN.

U N

N

K

W

O

N

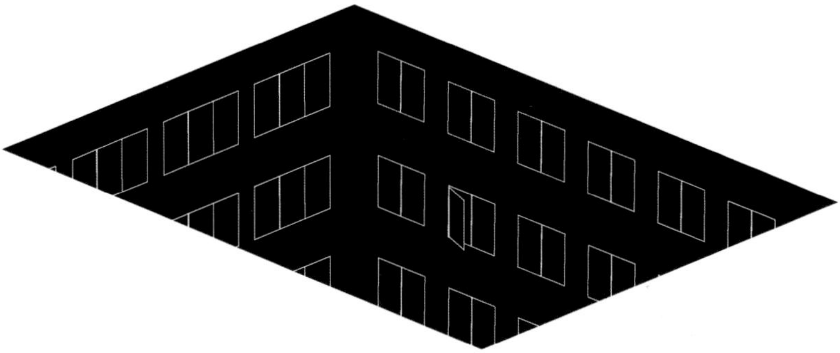

"DON'T BE AFRAID TO TRUST AN UNKNOWN FUTURE TO A **KNOWN** GOD[5]"

This is what FAITH is.

This is fighting the good fight of faith. This is pursuing God's best for your future.

TRUST IN GOD.

WE MUST

FIGHT

FOR OUR

FUTURE

WITH OUR

FAITH.

WE
EACH
HAVE A
FIGHTER
INSIDE
OF US.

What are we fighting for?

The hardest fight of our lives is not just about us.

YOU CAN’T AFFORD TO GIVE UP.

The fight of
your life is
for all the
people
you will be
able to help
after you
win it for
yourself.

We fight the battle to win

When we **win...**

we have a
battle story we
can tell!

Think of...

the people in your world
— and in your future —
that you will be able to
encourage because you
did not give up.

You can show them how
God went to work in your
life and how He is faithful
to go to work in their lives!

We are in this battle to WIN the battle!

We can win if we don't give up.

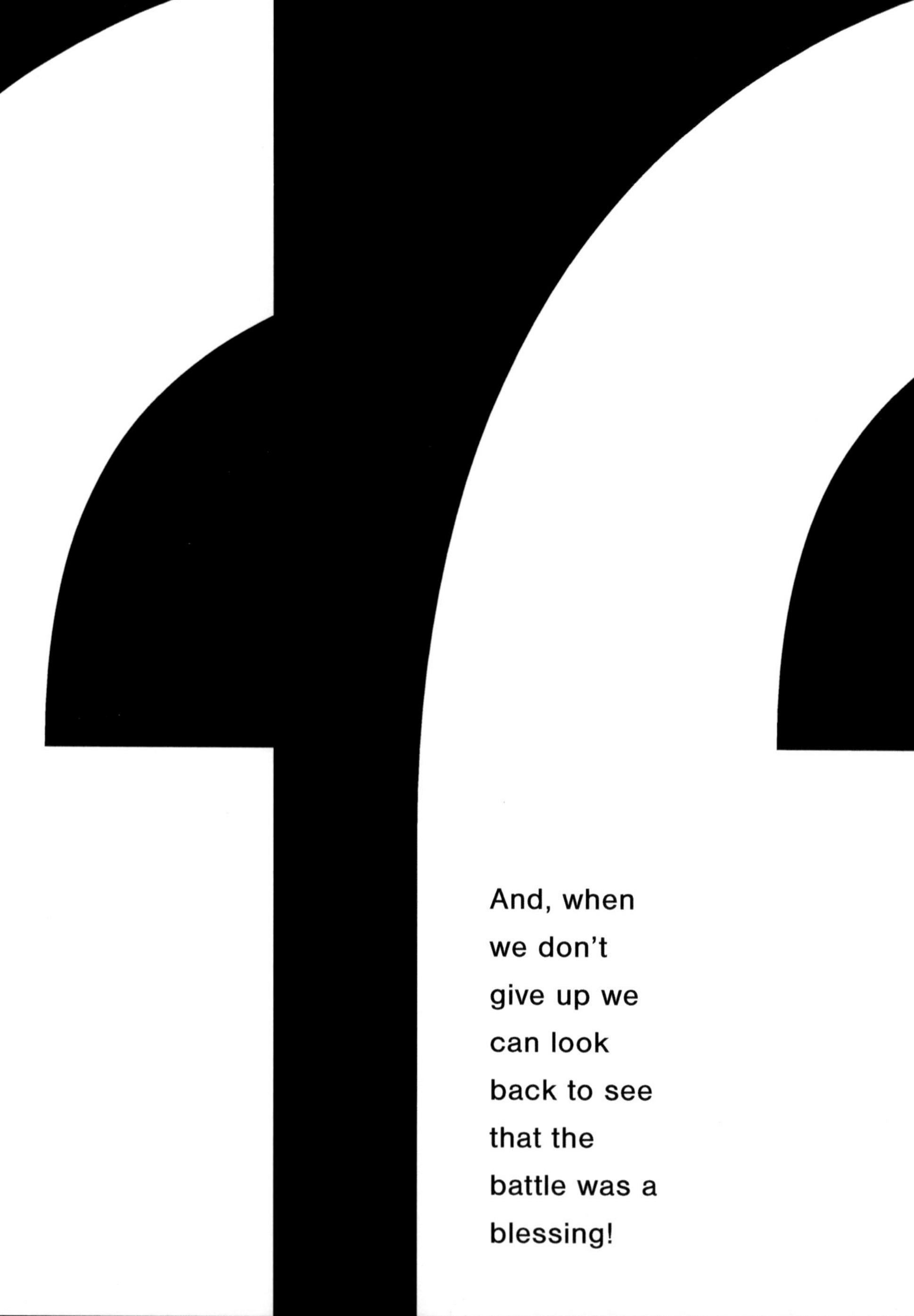

And, when we don't give up we can look back to see that the battle was a blessing!

When we get discouraged, remember who God says we are and how He says

WE WILL WIN THE FIGHT.

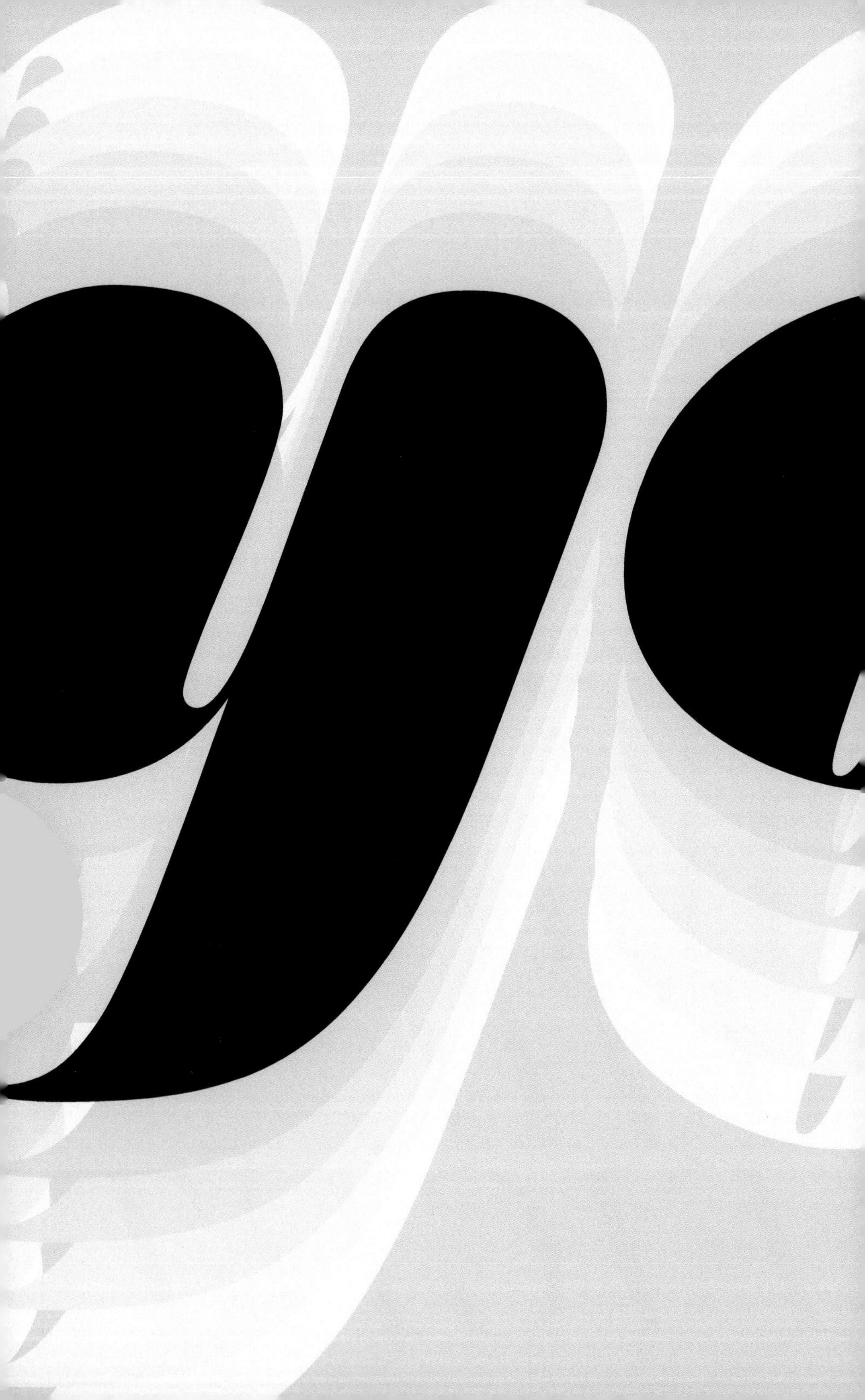

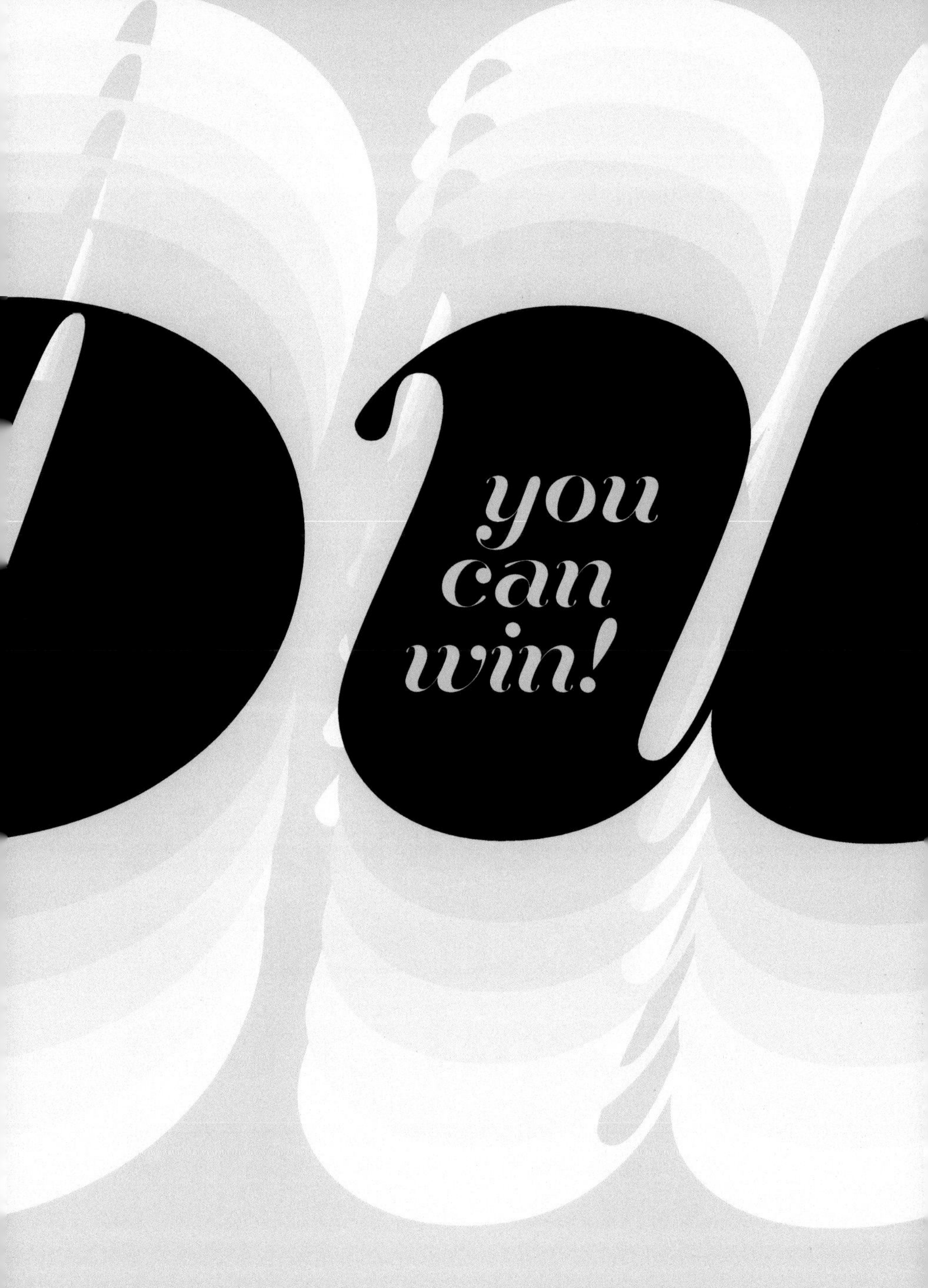
you
can
win!

Be the kind of person who pulls out the boxing gloves and compels yourself to stand in the mirror and say,

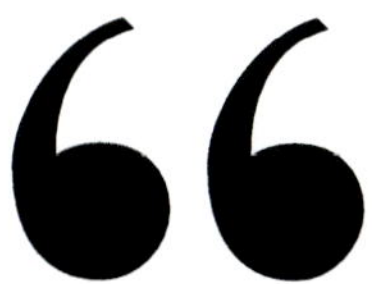

My best days are ahead of me... my battle is a blessing...

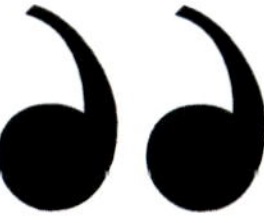

I will win this fight if I don't give up.

Put on the full Armor of God to help you stand your ground.

Put on the Belt of Truth and set your feet in God's peace. Put on the Breastplate of Righteousness and the Helmet of Salvation. Arm yourself with a Shield of Faith, and the Sword of the Spirit which is the word of God. [6]

In the fight for your life, your heavenly Father is in YOUR corner.

He believes in you!

It doesn't matter what anyone else has said for us or against us.

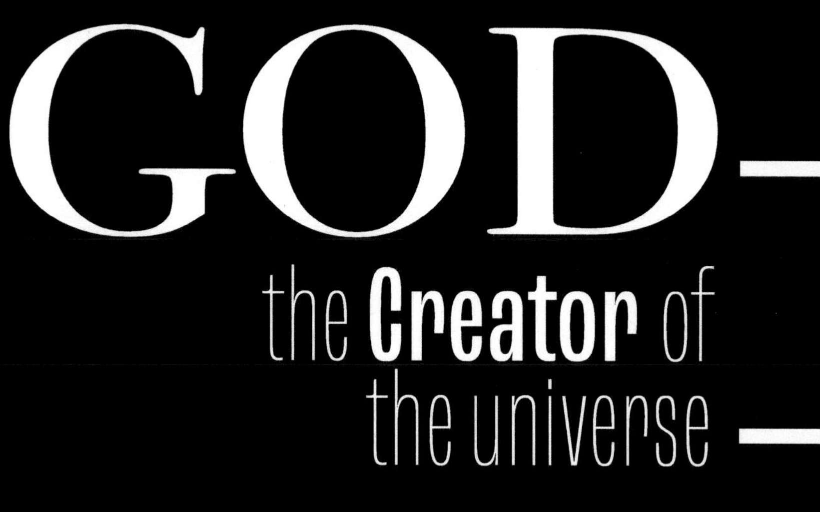

IS IN OUR CORNER!

God will NEVER miss one of our fights...

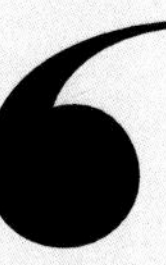

He already said, "**I will never leave you nor forsake you.**"[7] God has our back.

Whether we can see Him or not. Whether we can feel Him or not. God is with us and He is for us.

God has given you and me the power to overcome. He has given us the ability to win!

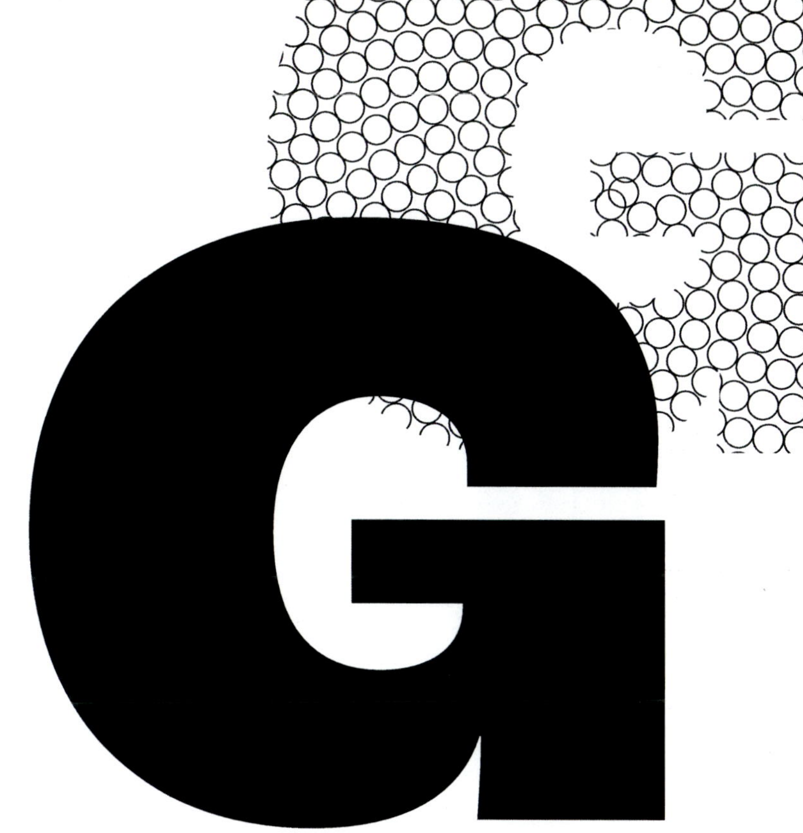

God

is greater than the enemy we are facing.

God is for you,

so who can be against you?[8]

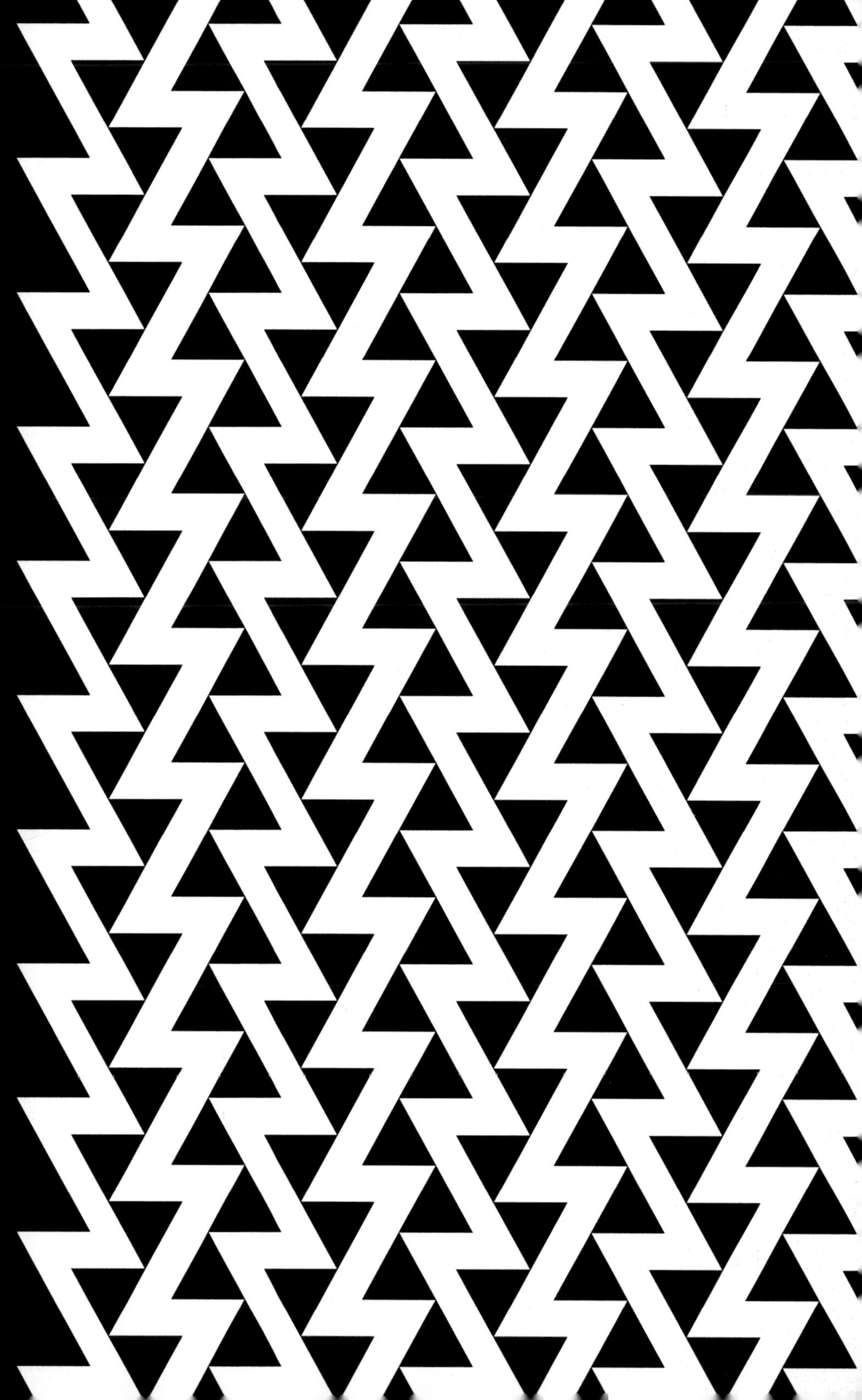

REMEMBER,

YOU ARE STRONG

You were born to fight.

CHOOSE TO FIGHT

THE **GOOD** FIGHT.

God believes in

YOU

NOW

it's your turn to

believe in
you.

End

	Page	
1	07	1 Timothy 6:12a NIV
2	16	John Maxwell quote
3	32	1 Thessalonians 5:17
4	51	Ephesians 4:29 TPT
5	59	Corrie Ten Boom quote
6	76-77	Ephesians 6:14-18 paraphrase
7	80	Hebrews 13:5 ESV
8	84-85	Romans 8:31 NIV

THE THANK YOU'S:

Thanks to God for turning my healing into hope so it can help someone else on the journey. And thank you Ryan, my husband, for being so supportive. I appreciate each of my family and friends who took some moments to move this project forward. Thank you to SpeakU Creative for bringing this very visual project to life. And, lastly, thank you, reader, for making it this far! I would love to hear your story, connect with me on social media or at JodiCameron.com and share your story with me!

Until next time,

-Jodi

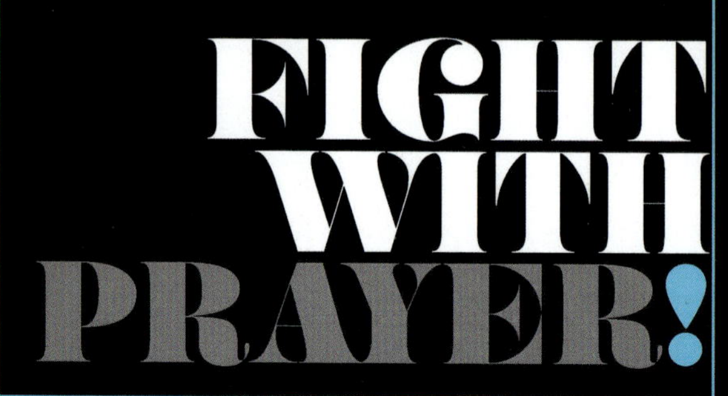

For a free 7-day devotional to up your prayer game, check out JodiCameron.com!

Let's Stay Connected.

Send me your fight stories on

JodiCameron.com